STAYING STRONG :
SIMPLE WAYS TO MAINTAIN THAT ERECTION

Godfrey Hunt

Table of Contents

Chapter 1

Erection, Size, and Dysfunction- No need to worry

How do erections happen?

Blood rushes in through the cavernosus arteries to fill the corpora cavernosa's blood vessels as they relax and widen. Erection results from the blood becoming trapped under intense pressure.

Stimulation of the senses and the mind triggers an erection. Nerve signals start to arouse the penis during sexual desire. The muscles of the corpora cavernosa relax in response to the brain and local nerve impulses, allowing blood to enter and fill the empty areas. An erection is produced when the blood causes pressure in the corpora cavernosa, which causes the penis to enlarge.

The tunica albuginea, a membrane that surrounds the corpora cavernosa, assists in keeping blood in the cavernosa, maintaining an erection. When the penile muscles contract, the blood flow is stopped and outflow channels are opened, which prevents erection from occurring.

Normal penis size

So, is there a typical penis size? A simple no is a response. Men come in a variety of sizes and forms. The majority of pens come in various sizes and styles. And they all have distinct appearances: they might be straight, curved, long, thick, thin, circumcised, or not. No, one is not superior to the other. Inside your pants, your penis typically hangs to one side.

A penis typically measures 6 to 13 centimetres in length when soft. Typically, an upright one measures between 7 and 17 centimetres long. 12 centimetres is roughly average. Compared to huge penises, smaller penises enlarge more when they are erect.

Measure your penis while it is upright and on the top side, which is the side closest to your belly.

Some quick facts to calm you down

You might or might not be surprised by erection-related facts, but they are undoubtedly fascinating. If you have a penis, you might be wondering whether the erections (or lack thereof) you're having are common. Here are a few erection-related facts that you might find interesting.

1. Those who have penises can get 3-5 erections each night.

Rapid eye movement (REM) sleep produces three to five erections every night for a person with a penis. It's not entirely clear why this occurs. However, a lot of doctors claim it's entirely normal.

2. Penises may fracture

You can indeed break your penis. However, it's not like a shattered bone; rather, the blood arteries in the penis burst, resulting in excruciating swelling. One-third of penile fracture cases, according to the National Health Service of the United Kingdom, are related to inverted sexual encounters.

3. In-the-womb erections are possible.

Although it hasn't been well investigated, it's thought that alterations in blood flow and contractions of the pelvic muscles may be responsible for fetal erections.

Fetal erections can happen anywhere between one to three times per hour on average during the third trimester of pregnancy, according to a 2020 review trusted Source. So you see, you have been having a boner before you were born!

4. The penis is not a bone or muscle.

Contrary to popular conception, neither a bone nor a muscle makes up the penis.

Instead, the penis is made up of three cylindrical chambers that resemble sponges and slowly fill with blood when you become excited.

A result of this is an increase in pressure that keeps blood from leaving the penis and resulting in an erection.

5. An average erection lasts between 5.1 and 5.5 inches.

The average male erection is thought to be over 6 inches long, but according to a significant assessment, it's more likely to be between 5.1 and 5.5 inches long.

Exercises and drugs cannot alter the size or length of your penis. So don't waste your money and time.

6. Youth might be affected by erectile dysfunction (ED).

Even though the risk of ED rises with age, it's a widespread issue that also affects a lot of young people.

Approximately 11% of sexually active males between the ages of 18 and 31 experienced mild ED, whereas only 3% said they had moderate-to-severe ED, according to a 2021 study.

7. ED may be an indication of a serious medical condition.

Sexual dysfunction may occasionally be a symptom of deeper problems. Any condition that affects the smooth muscle tissue, nerves, arteries, or hormone levels in the penis might cause ED.

Particular health issues can contribute to ED, including:

- diabetes and heart disease
- blood pressure is high.
- high levels of cholesterol

For this reason, it's crucial to consult your doctor if you have regular ED to make sure it's not brought on by any underlying medical conditions.

8. Orgasms don't necessitate erections

Yes, males who are unable to get erections can still experience orgasms.

Even without an erection, many men with ED can experience orgasm or ejaculation during sexual stimulation or intercourse.

9. Lifestyle decisions may increase your risk of developing ED.

You are more likely to develop ED if you experience stress, anxiety, smoke, or consume large amounts of alcohol.

A body mass index over 25, the use of specific drugs, and cycling for more than three hours per week are additional risk factors for ED.

Although most men occasionally have trouble achieving or maintaining an erection, if it happens regularly, if it's making you anxious, or if it's affecting your sexual relationships, you may want to speak with your doctor or go to a sexual health clinic.

10. ED stress might exacerbate the situation

Stress and anxiety can be brought on by having trouble getting or keeping an erection, and these emotions can make ED worse.

An ED that develops suddenly and is brought on by stress, depression, anxiety, or relationship issues are classified as psychogenic ED.

More on Erections

The penis grows larger and is briefly engorged with blood during an erection. It becomes stiff as a result of standing up and moving out from the body.

The cause is frequently sexual arousal, which can be brought on by something you see, feel, or even think about that makes you feel hot.

Additionally, erections might occur for no apparent reason. These sporadic erections are known as spontaneous erections.

Therefore, if you experience a stiffy while viewing a documentary about slugs, it's just a penis acting naturally and it's nothing to worry about.

It's also common to experience morning wood, whether or not you had a sex dream.

Flowing from our opening pages let us review the anatomy of the penis to understand how an erection functions.

The corpora cavernosa, which consists of two chambers, runs the length of your penis. Each one has a web of blood arteries that resembles sponges.

An erection is produced when those blood arteries relax and open, allowing blood to stream through and fill them.

The blood is trapped by a membrane around the corpora cavernosa, ensuring that your penis remains firm.

However, erections aren't only about the penis. Your brain also contributes.

Your brain sends messages to your penis when you become aroused, causing the muscles there to relax and permit blood flow.

However some lifestyle variables, like being exhausted, stressed out, or intoxicated can make it challenging for you to erect.

Erectile dysfunction can also be brought on by specific drugs and illnesses.

An erection can, however, be uncomfortable in some circumstances.

A good illustration of this is erection brought about by pee. They occur because your penis is made to prevent you from wetting yourself. It's quite wonderful. You'll feel the burn if you try to urinate while still hard.

To engage in penetrating sex, you need to have an erection.

Although you are not required to have penetrative sex if you don't want to, you must at least be somewhat hard to get it in there, whether there be a vagina or anus.

Without an erection, penetration resembles pushing rope.One approach is that the penis is made to lose an erection after you ejaculate.

When it comes to the ideal number of erections, there is no set formula.

Everybody is different, but men with penises typically have 11 erections per day and three to five more at night.

Your age, hormone levels, and lifestyle are just a few of the many variables that may have an impact on how frequently you become hard.

Being at ease and letting yourself become aroused are the keys to getting an erection.

Sexual stimulation ought to be enjoyable. Erections shouldn't make you feel bad or uncomfortable.

What's the verdict?

Erections occur frequently and are a normal component of having a penis. Even though they are annoying when they arise unexpectedly, having them is a sign of health.

They may primarily be there to facilitate penetration, but there is no pressure.

Chapter 2

Calm, Easy and good Diet does it: kill the anxiety

It's typical to feel a bit anxious before or during sex. Perhaps you're dating someone new or you're just a little on edge about making sure the other person gets the most pleasure possible.

However, performance anxiety can become an issue if it keeps you from wanting to have sex or when it interferes with your ability to enjoy sex. It can become so bad that erectile dysfunction or early ejaculation result.

You can have a satisfying sexual experience, and we're here to make it happen! For more information on what triggers sex anxiety and, more importantly, how to unwind during sex, continue reading.

What Leads to Sexual Panic?

The worry that your performance won't be up to par during sex is known as sexual performance anxiety. This kind of anxiousness not only compromises your mental health but also, let's face it, disrupts your general quality of life.

The most worrying aspect of sexual anxiety is that it can also result in erectile dysfunction or early ejaculation, in addition to making for unremarkable sexual encounters and difficulty with pleasure.

You may experience sexual performance anxiety for several reasons. The questions you might be concerned about before and during intercourse provide proof of some of the most prevalent worries. They could consist of:

- Can I expect to have an erection?

- Am I ejaculating too early?

- Am I attractive to my partner?

- How much penis do I have?

- Will my partner be satisfied?

- Will my companion experience orgasm?

Men who have poor body image may also experience anxiety during sexual activity. One-third of males with erectile dysfunction in a study of male military personnel under the age of 40 had an obsession with their genitalia and their body image.

Some guys may have anxiety related to sexual performance after watching porn. Comparisons between real-life experiences and those shown in pornography can make people feel inadequate. So my advice; porn hurts if you understand what I mean.

Your body has physical effects when you have sex-related anxiety and find it difficult to unwind. The sympathetic nervous system is activated by anxiety, which causes blood vessels to contract and release the stress chemicals cortisol, norepinephrine, and epinephrine.

What is the unfavourable outcome of this biological process? It gets more difficult to achieve and maintain an erection. This makes having sex much harder and less enjoyable.

According to one study, sexual performance anxiety is one of the factors most strongly associated with both male and female erectile dysfunction. (And for women, a lack of relaxation and sexual anxiousness can hurt when having sex.)

Anxiety about sexual performance occasionally goes away by itself. For instance, if it's brought on by being with a new person, it can fade away once you get used to your relationship.

You must determine the cause of your sex anxiety, though, if it persists. The most effective course of treatment will be chosen once the cause of the anxiety is understood.

Here are some of the most popular ways to get to bed earlier:

Therapy

Both sex therapy and cognitive behavioural therapy (CBT) are frequently employed to alleviate sexual performance anxiety. You will discuss the causes of your anxiety and develop coping mechanisms in treatment.

CBT is predicated on the notion that negative thought patterns and behaviours can contribute to psychological issues. In CBT, a person learns to identify skewed thinking and is provided with problem-solving techniques to deal with challenging circumstances.

You can go to sex therapy alone or with a partner. An expert in sex therapy may start by inquiring about a client's sexual history, sex education, and sex-related attitudes.

Speak with a healthcare provider about your treatment choices if your ED or sexual performance anxiety is interfering with your ability to enjoy sex.

Treatments for premature ejaculation

You're not alone if you worry that you'll ejaculate before you should. According to research, worry about sexual performance is significantly related to worries about early ejaculation.

Applying an anaesthetizing lotion or spray to the penis is another typical remedy for ejaculating too fast. This helps the penis become less sensitive so you can wait longer between ejaculations. You should be able to find a good one.

Sex should be enjoyed at, the end of the story. Enjoy your time in bed. And if you experience nervousness, you are undoubtedly not taking full advantage of your sexual opportunities.

There are techniques to help you unwind during sex, regardless of what's causing your worry - whether it's early ejaculation, worries about erectile issues, or simply the fact that you're with someone new and want to impress them.

To profit from the health advantages that healthy sexual experiences can provide and, yes, get your sex life back, speak with a healthcare provider as soon as possible if you believe that medicine will help you most.

If you notice any self-criticism at all, then ignore it as background noise, and go back to concentrating on providing and receiving pleasure.

Ideally, discuss your feelings regarding your sexual experiences with your spouse in-between practice sessions. That sexual activity may be delightful even when things don't go perfectly can hopefully be reinforced by such chats, as long as you keep the pleasure in mind rather than your judgment and fear.

However, ED doesn't necessarily have a physical cause. ED can be caused by a variety of reasons, including:abrupt changes in habit, increasing daily stress, major dietary or nutritional changes, and mental health disorders including depression

This is why it's a good idea to consult a doctor whenever you suspect ED symptoms are present. A doctor can identify your symptoms more precisely and rule out any additional causes for them.

The only way to express how you're feeling and what you're going through to your spouse is through conversation.

Use this opportunity to bring up any worries, dissatisfaction, or even boredom you may be feeling about your current sexual life.

Here are some ideas to get a good conversation started:

Your partner or relationship may not necessarily be the cause of your dissatisfaction with your sexual life. Keep your thoughts from straying too far in either direction. Try to reassure your companion as best you can. This coupling probably won't end after talking about your sexual life; you could just need something new to keep things interesting.

We frequently pick up sexual practices from the media we watch. This covers both positive and unfavourable portrayals of sexual behaviour. Recognize that you or your partner may not want what you believe sex should be.

Timing is crucial. Concentration is appropriate right now. During a sensitive topic, you don't want to take the chance of making your spouse feel ignored.

Change things up in the bedroom.

Try to liven up your diet or lifestyle before making any long-term or dramatic changes.

Fresh positions to tighten the anal or vaginal area, have your partner keep their legs closer together while you enter or perform the move from behind while lying on your side or with them on their hands and knees.

The penis, clitoris, or anus can be stimulated with the help of handheld vibrators, penis rings, butt plugs, and anal beads. Use caution when using these things, and clean them after each use.

To create excitement, use your tongues to create erogenous zones on one another's genitalia or other body parts.

Do you have a straight partner but have only engaged in vaginal sex? Ask your spouse whether they'd be willing to peg you with a toy or try anal on you. Make sure you have enough lubricant! You don't want any off putting situations now.

Role-playing. Create a scenario or take on a persona to help you create an enticing tale about your sexual encounter.

Pay less attention to sexual performance. Instead, put more effort into figuring out what kind of contact makes you feel the happiest.

And one of the secrets to maintaining regular, healthy erections is blood flow to the penis.

The following foods may be helpful:

According to a 1993 study by trusted Source, fruits rich in antioxidants and anthocyanins, like blueberries, can aid to protect body tissues and reduce your risk of heart disease. A 2019 study found that foods high in vitamin B12, such as fermented soy-based tempeh, can promote other biological processes that enhance erectile health.

Oatmeal and other foods high in L-arginine have been shown in a 2003 study to enhance blood flow and relax muscles.

Consume fewer fried, greasy, and processed foods.

According to a 1994 study, eating a diet high in fatty, fried, or processed foods may raise your risk of developing illnesses that can damage your sexual health and general well-being.

These circumstances include:

- diabetes high blood pressure and heart disease

It might be useful to:
Replace high-fat dairy products with low-fat alternatives, such as yoghurt and milk.
Choose whole-grain or oat cereals rather than processed cereals.
Keep salad greens and other quick-to-prepare veggies and grains like quinoa on hand if you're typically strapped for time.
Create a quick, wholesome dinner using these basic whole ingredients, or prepare a few meals in advance.
The Mediterranean diet is an example.
The Mediterranean diet may help with several underlying issues that may contribute to erectile dysfunction, according to some 2017 studies.
This diet may be helpful:
Reduce cholesterol; boost antioxidants
boosting L-arginine levels enhances blood flow.
Start by eating more of the following if you aren't ready to switch or wish to do so gradually:
such as carrots, spinach, and kale

Nuts and seeds like almonds, walnuts, and sunflower seeds, as well as fruits like apples, bananas, and grapes

legumes, such as lentils, beans, and peanuts

tubers such as yams and potatoes

eggs from birds such as chicken and turkey

dairy items like Greek yoghurt and cheese

avocados and extra-virgin olive oil are examples of healthy fats.

Reduce your alcohol consumption.

In a 2007 study, heavy alcohol use was linked to an increased incidence of sexual dysfunction.

Usually, one or two beers won't hurt. It might even assist to reduce your risk of erectile dysfunction, according to a 2018 review from trusted Source.

However, there is a direct link between your alcohol consumption and the frequency of your sex performance problems.

Please consume more caffeine.

Love tea or coffee? Great! Caffeine may increase blood flow and relax the muscles that help you get and maintain an erection, according to a 2005 assessment.

Just black coffee, unsweetened tea, and caffeinated beverages without sugars are what you should aim for.

Get 20 minutes or more a day of moderate exercise.

According to a 2013 research erectile dysfunction may suffer from physical inactivity.

Just 20 minutes of exercise each day can help with weight management and improved circulation, two important aspects of general erectile health.

Make time to go for a little stroll or jog, or think about performing the following exercises in your home:

However, be mindful of how much time you spend cycling.

According to some 2015 research, riding can cause ED because it puts strain on the blood vessels and nerves in your pelvic area.

To determine whether there is a connection, more study is required.

Consider purchasing a seat that relieves some of the pressure on your perineum, where the pressure may do the most harm if you frequently cycle to work or just for enjoyment.

Ensure that you receive enough sleep.

A 2005 study by a trusted Source found that a lack of sleep, particularly as a result of sleep apnea and other sleep problems, is associated with a higher chance of developing ED.

According to a 2019 study, not getting enough sleep may also increase your risk of atherosclerosis, or artery plaque.

Your circulation may be impacted by this, which will make getting and maintaining an erection more challenging.

Here are some suggestions to help you obtain your recommended 6 to 8 hours every night:

At least an hour before going to bed, turn off all screens, including your phone, computer, and TV.

After about 6 p.m., stay away from caffeine-containing beverages.

Any midday naps should be kept to no more than one hour.

Try to have a consistent bedtime and wake-up time each day.

One hour before going to bed, think about taking a melatonin supplement.

Keep the temperature in your bedroom around 70 degrees Fahrenheit (21 degrees Celsius).

Make every effort to reduce or better control your stress.

According to research, psychological issues including stress and worry are frequently to blame for ED.

Play some music.

You can disperse essential oils or light an aromatherapy candle.

Write your thoughts down in a journal.

A comedy show or amusing movie can make you laugh.

Try to reduce your nicotine consumption.

Blood vessels can be harmed by nicotine and other compounds found in vaporizers, cigarettes, cigars, and other goods. Reduce the effectiveness of nitric oxide

When you're erect, nitric oxide widens your blood vessels, facilitating easier blood flow.

It may be harder to get into and maintain an erect posture if its effectiveness is compromised.

Focus more on what makes you feel good than on how well you're performing sexually if you want to lower your nervousness about performing.

Here, communication is essential. Maintaining the intimacy and trust necessary for a good sexual relationship can be accomplished by openly discussing any anger, resentment, humiliation, or unresolved difficulties.

Your sexual performance may also be impacted by low testosterone levels. If you experience any of the following, consult a doctor:

- lower volume of semen
- unusual baldness
- chronic exhaustion
- having difficulties concentrating
- having memory issues losing muscular mass

- abnormal accumulation of fat, particularly in the chest (gynecomastia)

If necessary, your doctor can recommend treatment and order certain blood tests.

You might also be wondering "why isn't my erection as powerful as it once was?"

It's rather typical to experience a decline in our sexual health as we age. Older males are also significantly more likely to have ED.

The degree of your overall arousal may also influence how strong your erection is. It's important to take into account any recent alterations to your relationships or way of life that could be impacting your arousal.

Because the penis typically ceases to be erect after ejaculation, this length of time is shortened for someone who reaches orgasm swiftly.

An erection can persist significantly longer for persons who "last longer" during sex or have a prolonged sexual session.

However, an erection typically lasts for 7 to 13 minutes during a sexual session.

However, seek emergency medical assistance if your erection persists for more than four hours. You might be having priapism. The inability of blood to exit the penis is a serious medical condition. It may result in severe or long-lasting harm if

Chapter 3

Declutter your Mind

Understanding why you have these thoughts is crucial before beginning any of the techniques to stop your negative thinking.

We'll discuss four of these reasons for mental clutter in this section.

Cause#1:Daily stress

The main cause of why so many people experience life-overwhelm is excessive stress. The stress brought on by physical clutter, an abundance of information, and the unending choices these items demand can lead to a variety of mental health problems like melancholy, panic attacks, and generalized anxiety.

According to the American Psychological Association, when you combine this stress with the real worries and concerns in your life, you may experience sleep issues, muscle discomfort, headaches, chest pain, recurrent infections, and stomach and intestinal illnesses (not to mention other health issues) and particularly, erectile dysfunction.

Numerous research has established a link between stress and bodily issues.

Before he suffered a full-blown panic attack on live television, ABC News anchor Dan Harris, who is also the author of the book 10% Happier, didn't realize how the stress of mental overload was affecting him.

He had been concerned and depressed because of his difficult and competitive job, which had taken him to the front lines of Afghanistan, Israel, Palestine, and Iraq. He used recreational drugs to treat his internal pain, which led to the on-air attack.

Dan's doctor visit ended with a wake-up call regarding his mental health. "As I sat there in his office, the sheer enormity of my mindlessness started to sink in—from hurtling headlong into war zones without considering the psychological repercussions to using drugs for a synthetic squirt of replacement," he writes in a post on the ABC website.

Don't let stress get to you, it will negatively affect your sex life.

Cause #2: The Choice Paradox

In terms of mental health, the freedom of choice, which is prized in free societies, can have a diminishing point of return. The term "paradox of choice," which was coined by psychologist Barry Schwartz, sums up his research showing that having more options causes people to feel more anxious, uncertain, paralyzed, and unsatisfied. Although having more options may result in objectively superior outcomes, you won't be delighted with them.

Take a straightforward trip to the grocery shop. The average store carried 42,214 goods in 2014, according to the Food Marketing Institute. Choosing the best brand of yoghurt or the ideal gluten-free crackers now takes at least as much time as what might have once been a 10-minute trip to get the necessities.

The most common item in most wardrobes, buying a pair of jeans will present you with a seemingly limitless number of options. slouchy fit? shoe cut? Skinny?

broad leg? vintage cleaning Knot fly? Zipper? Even a small purchase can cause you to become extremely anxious.

To reduce emotions of decision overload, Steve Jobs, Mark Zuckerberg, and even President Obama decided to restrict their outfit options. The president stated the reasoning behind his constrained outfit choices in a story by Michael Lewis for Vanity Fair:

You'll see that I only wear grey or blue suits, remarked Obama. "I want to make fewer decisions. I don't want to decide what I'm going to eat or wear. because I need to make too many other decisions. Put yourself in situations that make you take fewer decisions, it concomitantly clears your mind for better sex life.

Cause #3: Information Overload

We have a lot of items in our houses that we never use, such as clothes, unread novels, toys, and electronic devices. Our email inboxes are bursting at the seams. Our phones are displaying notifications like "You need more storage," and our PCs are cluttered.

We have become such gadget slaves that we would rather have the instant gratification of instant information or entertainment than real-world relationships and experiences.

Being a mass consumer of goods and data is now simpler than ever because of the constant flow of information and accessibility to technology. We can easily order anything online and have it delivered to our home, from a book to a motorboat.

We're stuffing our homes with unnecessary items and spending all of our free time reading tweets, updates, articles, blog posts, and cat videos. Around us, information and things are accumulating, but we feel powerless to do anything about it.

Our time and productivity are both wasted by all of this unnecessary information, which also causes reactive, anxious, and pessimistic thoughts.

Like: "My Facebook friend seems to be leading a contented life. My life is terrible.

Should I purchase the FitBit and begin monitoring my health so I don't pass away too soon?

Oh crap, I completely forgot about that webinar on "How to Make a Million Before You're 30"—what if they revealed something crucial?

Everything appears urgent and important. Responses to all emails and texts are required. Every new gadget or contraption needs to be bought. This keeps us distracted from the people around us and the emotions inside of us, continuously riled up and preoccupied with unimportant things.

We frequently believe that we are too busy ingesting new things and information to have time to simplify. But eventually, all of this activity is wearing us out mentally and emotionally. We analyze, ruminate, and worry ourselves to the breaking point as we try to process everything that is being presented to us.

How did we come to forget the principles and goals in life that used to keep us centred and sane? How can we handle it? We are unable to travel back in time and abandon technology. We can't give up everything we have in this world and live in a cave. We need to find a means to survive in the present day without going insane.

Some of the anxiety and negative thinking can be relieved by organizing our belongings and spending less time on technology.

But there are still many reasons for us to get bogged down in regret, worry, and other negative thoughts.

We fret about a variety of things, including terrorism, politics, pain from the past, our uncertain futures, and our health, jobs, kids, relationships, economy, and appearance. If we didn't have that constant voice in our heads stirring things up, we wouldn't suffer from our thoughts about these things and would be happier right now.

The long and short of this is that our sex life takes a hit. What do you want to do about it.

Some Solutions

You probably don't think about your breathing very often, even though you take about 20,000 breaths per day. Your brain automatically modifies your breathing to meet your body's needs. When you're climbing stairs or going for a run, you don't have to think, "I better breathe deeper and harder to get more oxygen to my muscles." It just happens.

It is the responsibility of sensors in your brain, blood vessels, muscles, and lungs to adjust your breathing to your body's changing needs. However, you have the authority to do so whenever you desire. Breathing can be slowed down, changed from the chest to the abdomen, and even made shallower or deeper.

The first indication that our thoughts are stressful and overwhelming is frequently a change in breathing. We may breathe quickly or become short of breath when we are stressed, depressed, rushed, or upset. Poor, shallow breathing is also a result of our contemporary lifestyles and work environments.

In Peace of Mindfulness: Everyday Rituals to Conquer Anxiety and Claim Unlimited

Inner Peace, written by Barrie: Unfortunately, we spend most of the day sitting still, so we don't need to breathe deeply like our ancestors did when they were out hunting, gathering, farming, or doing other manual labour. We have gotten into the habit of short, shallow breathing when we are slouched over our desks or watching TV on the couch.

When we're hurried and pressed for time, we breathe quickly and nervously. Our bodies constrict when we're under stress, anxious, or preoccupied with a problem, and we hunch forward with our heads bowed, arms clasped, and muscles tense.

2. "Meditation is not a technique for quieting the mind. It's a technique for gaining access to the silence that is already present but hidden by the average person's daily 50,000 thoughts. According to Deeksha Chopra to meditate, you don't need to be a Buddhist, mystic, or ex-hippie carrying a crystal. Anyone can benefit from meditation and use it as a tool to clear their

mind, regardless of their spiritual or religious affiliation or lack thereof.

The thought of sitting still in the lotus position and emptying your mind may be off-putting if you've never meditated or are unfamiliar with it. But don't let the cliches about cave dwellers who practice meditation stop you from trying it.

Dan Harris writes in his book 10% Happier, "Meditation suffers from a towering PR problem... But if you can get past the cultural baggage, you'll discover that meditation is just brain exercise.

Since it has been around for so long, meditation has its roots in the ancient Buddhist, Hindu, and Chinese traditions. There are many different types of meditation, but they all start with the same steps: sitting still, concentrating on your breath, and ignoring any outside distractions.

Depending on the method of meditation practised and the desired results of the practitioner, different goals can be set for meditation. For this article, we recommend meditation as a tool to assist you in developing mental discipline and thought control, both while you are sitting in meditation and when you are not.

The advantages of meditation carry over to your daily life, assisting you in reducing anxiety and overthinking as well as offering a variety of health advantages, which we'll go over below.

Simply practising meditation can help you become successful at it. You will develop your skills and learn how the mental, physical, and emotional advantages grow over time by committing to meditating every day.

Chapter 4

Your Weigh and Self Image are Key

What Does Weight Have to Do with Better Sex?

Your libido does suffer if you are overweight. Small adjustments, though, can ignite your sex drive.

However, cultural messages also continue to convey to us that anyone larger than a size 6 should refrain from succumbing to sexual seduction. Being overweight and attractive don't go together like oil and water. That potent message can quickly dampen even the most robust libido for those already dealing with weight and image problems.

Martin Binks, PhD, a clinical psychologist and director of behavioural health at Duke University's Diet and Fitness Center in Durham, North Carolina, says: "Unfortunately, people are internalizing society's definition of what it takes to be involved in sex, particularly the body shape — there are societal biases out there that are influencing us on an individual level and not in a good way."

However, it appears that cultural messages don't tell the complete story. According to recent studies, some physical issues that are associated with obesity may also have an impact on sex desire, which would further reduce an overweight person's desire. The good news is that you can alter your body and your perspective on it to improve your libido. One can:

To activate sex hormones, reduce weight by even 10 pounds.

Consume more nutrient-rich foods to lower cholesterol and blood sugar.

Your workouts should focus on promoting blood flow to the pelvic region.

Start reading a seductive book and accept your body at any size.

Consider yourself sensual;

How do I start? Determine the potential physical and mental barriers to having a satisfying sexual life by starting there.

Up to 30% of obese adults seeking assistance with weight reduction, according to recent research by Binks and his colleagues at Duke, report issues with sex drive, desire, performance, or all three. According to the most recent studies, these issues are frequently linked to physical conditions that coexist with obesity.

According to Andrew McCollough, MD, director of sexual health and male infertility at NYU Medical Center in New York, "Medical conditions like high cholesterol and insulin resistance [an early indicator of type 2 diabetes] do have the ability to impact sexual performance, which in turn impacts desire, particularly in men."

McCollough claims that impotence or erectile dysfunction is frequently the outcome of both disorders because they have the potential to cause the tiny arteries in the penis to close off, particularly when vessel-clogging fatty deposits start to accumulate.

According to McCollough, a man who struggles to get an erection would soon lose his desire for sex.

Poor blood flow is not just a concern for men who have sex issues. According to research, a woman's weight has an impact on her desire and sex drive.

According to Susan Kellogg, PhD, director of sexual medicine at the Pelvic and Sexual Health Institute of Graduate Hospital in Philadelphia, "we are starting to see that the width of the blood vessels leading to the clitoris [the area of the vagina most closely related to sexual response] in women are affected by the same kind of blockages that impact blood flow to the penis."

According to Kellogg, when this occurs, a woman's physiology is far less receptive, and a decrease in desire follows quickly.

Further complicating situations for both sexes: Your levels of a natural substance called SHBG to increase with body fat percentage (short for sex hormone binding globulin). Because it binds to the sex hormone testosterone, it is suitably named. According to medical experts, testosterone is less available to enhance desire the more it is linked to SHBG.

Simple Modifications to Increase Your Sex Drive

How can your physical fitness for sex be improved? Plenty. According to experts, decreasing as little as 10 pounds can frequently release testosterone and increase your love life nearly immediately.

Better news still. Even if you don't lose weight, making the same dietary adjustments that lower blood sugar and cholesterol, such as switching to a low-fat diet and eating more fruits and vegetables, can improve your sex drive.

"I've observed that very often when patients start to take better care of themselves, they also report a significant increase in their interest in sex," says Binks. "I think participation in a healthy lifestyle helps, even if you don't lose the extra pounds."

Additionally, Kellogg claims that activities meant to improve circulation to the genitals rather than for weight loss can have a significant impact, especially on women.

According to Kellogg, any exercise that improves blood flow to the big muscle groups in the thighs, buttocks, and pelvis, such as yoga, brisk walking, or cycling for 20 minutes three times a week, will also help hydrate the genitalia. She claims that increased lubrication, better arousal, and improved orgasmic function are the outcomes. Finally, there is a resurgence of sexual desire.

In addition, Kellogg advises ladies to think about adding 20 minutes of light sensual reading three times a week to their sexy workout. Here, it's important to put the spotlight back on sex to increase drive and desire.

"Grocery shopping, PTA meetings, or cleaning are hardly particularly sexy activities. Number of your size or shape, if that occupies all of your thoughts, there is no room for sex-related ideas "affirms Kellogg.

"When a woman simply feels better and feels gorgeous, weight becomes less of a problem," she claims.

You'll be sexy if you think sexy.

Which brings up the possibility of what's going on in your thoughts. For some people, resolving bodily issues is all it takes to ignite their desire. Others still feel that it falls short.

According to experts, having a negative body image is one of the largest barriers to enjoying sex at any size. They warn you against sleeping alone in a double bed if people can't accept your size and weight.

In a way, society almost tells us that you have to hate your body before you can improve it, according to Binks. "There is this idea out there that if you accept your body and your weight that it's somehow going to take away your motivation to change the way you look," she says.

He claims that this mindset frequently makes overweight people feel so self-conscious about how they appear that desire is completely suppressed.

Abby Aronowitz, PhD, a psychologist and expert on body image, concurs. "Giving up self-consciousness to fully experience the moment is the height of sexuality. It's pretty impossible to enjoy the moment, much less be there for your partner, if you're worried about this bulge, that bulge, or how your butt looks from every angle "author of Your Final Diet, Aronowitz.

Although both men and women can be harmed by body image, researchers concur that women are more affected than men. Kellogg claims that if a woman's body image deviates from the "average," even if she has a loving spouse, she may still think of herself as sexually unappealing.

Even if her boyfriend tells her she is, a woman who doesn't perceive herself to be sexually attractive will not believe that she is, according to Kellogg.

Still, lacking in sexual desire? Get support.

Even while simple lifestyle adjustments and positive self-talk can significantly increase motivation and desire, professional image counselling may be necessary if you still struggle with this.

"Regardless of your size, obtaining treatment that works toward boosting self-esteem will reflect in your desire for sex and your capacity to find sexual fulfilment if you are someone who has negative views about your body image," says Binks. Your primary care physician is frequently the best place to start. However, experts advise not to be afraid to seek out a counsellor with experience in body image and weight concerns if you feel you require more specific assistance.

The most important thing to keep in mind is that, despite research showing that up to 30% of overweight persons experience sexual issues, Binks points out that up to 70% of them are doing just fine, and you can too.

The secret, according to Aronowitz, is to "let your sexuality and sensuality thrive inside the body you have" rather than buying into society's ideal of ideal sexual body.

What impact does body weight have on sex drive?

Your body weight might have a significant impact on your sex drive. You can try to deny it all you want, but how you feel about yourself can have a big impact on your sexual performance and desire. According to studies, having a depleted sex desire can result from being overweight. Here are several ways that your weight may have an impact on your libido in light of that.

Body weight gain can increase globulin, which lowers the levels of the sex hormone testosterone. Your libido and sexual impulses may decline significantly as a result of a dip in the sex hormone, which can affect your sex drive.

Women's sex drives and body image and confidence have frequently been correlated in research. People who are overweight often experience severe insecurity and discomfort. People who are healthy and fit, on the other hand, exude an aura of confidence. Having said that, a lot of your sexual performance is influenced by how you see yourself.

Men who are obese frequently have trouble arousing their sex drives. According to several experts, obesity reduces men's testosterone levels, which results in less

sexual desire. This can occasionally cause men to experience erectile dysfunction. Men who are overweight or obese are more likely to have heart disease, diabetes, and high cholesterol, all of which might increase the likelihood that they will experience erectile Additionally, being overweight might cause blood vessels to constrict, which improves blood flow to the genitalia. Therefore, both men and women have trouble attaining a climax without appropriate blood flow. This frequently results in a declining sex drive.
Your physical makeup facilitates and aids in the fulfilment of your sexual dreams. Your sexual movements may likely be limited if you are obese. Nevertheless, it might be off-putting and can ruin your desire for sex.

9 798357 929150